THE HEALING TRIBUNE

THE CAUSE OF DISEASE MADE SIMPLE

THE CAUSE AND SOLUTION FOR BREAST CANCER REVEALED

BOOK 4

DANNY CARROLL

RECALL PUBLISHING

I would like to dedicate this book to the late Dr. Ryke Geerd Hamer. I very sadly did not get to meet Dr. Hamer before he died in 2017. Without a doubt, Dr. Hamer was the greatest medical mind to ever be put on this earth. He singlehandedly unraveled the biological code, and then spent the rest of his life being persecuted for his medical discoveries.

I would also like to dedicate this book to Helmut Pilhar. Helmut was Dr. Hamer's chosen lecturer to spread Germanic Healing Knowledge. Helmut was the tip of the spear and dedicated his life to teaching GHk. He very sadly passed away on 31 August 2022.

May their souls rest in eternal peace.

CONTENTS

ISBN Issued in print and electronic formats.

ISBN 978-1-915838-04-9 (eBook)

ISBN 978-1-915838-05-6 (Paperback)

ISBN 978-1-915838-06-3 (Hardback)

ISBN 978-1-915838-07-0 (Audiobook)

Disclaimer:

Please note: The author of this book is not a medical doctor. The information contained in this book is for educational purposes only. All effort has been made to present accurate, up-to-date, complete, and reliable information. No warranties of any kind are stated or implied. Readers acknowledge that the author is not engaging in the rendering of medical, legal, financial, or professional advice. Please consult a licensed professional before attempting any techniques outlined in this book.

Under no circumstances will any legal responsibility be held against the publisher or author for any damages, reparations, or monetary loss due to the information contained within this book, neither directly nor indirectly. The content within this book has been derived from multiple sources, including details of the author's own healing experiences.

By reading this book, the reader agrees that under no circumstances will the author or publisher be held responsible for any losses, direct or indirect, which are incurred as a result of implementing the information contained in this book, including, but not limited to, — errors, omissions, or inaccuracies. You are responsible for your own choices, actions, and results.

THE HEALING TRIBUNE

Sign up to claim a Free 400+ page eBook
That includes the 'CAUSES' of nearly all known diseases with over 500 case studies.

Plus, a **FREE One-Year Course** of 6–7-minute MP3 daily classes to start learning Germanic Healing Knowledge.

You'll also receive my free monthly installments of

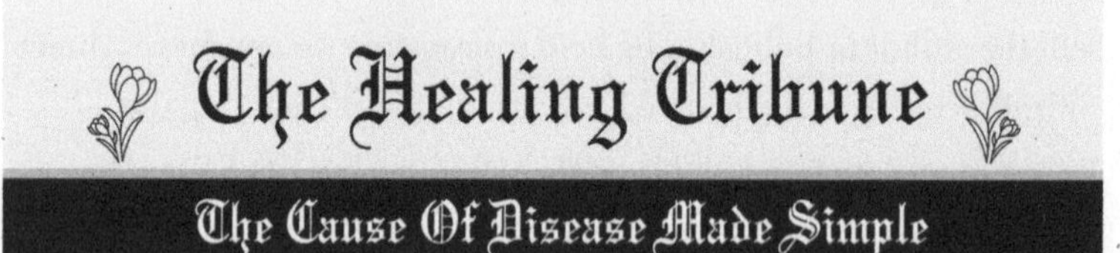

Unsubscribe anytime. Keep your free gift.

Sign up at https://danny-carroll.com

INTRODUCTION

Welcome to the fourth edition of "The Healing Tribune." Today, I will discuss breast cancer. I selected this for the fourth edition of The Healing Tribune because it is one of the leading causes of cancer deaths in women.

This information is provided by **Breastcancer.org.**

About 1 in 8 U.S. women (about 13%) will develop invasive breast cancer over the course of their lifetime.

In 2022, an estimated 287,850 new cases of invasive breast cancer are expected to be diagnosed in women in the U.S., along with 51,400 new cases of non-invasive (in situ) breast cancer.

About 2,710 new cases of invasive breast cancer are expected to be diagnosed in men in 2022. A man's lifetime risk of breast cancer is about 1 in 833.

Breast cancer is the most commonly diagnosed cancer among American women. In 2022, it's estimated that about 30% of newly diagnosed cancers in women will be breast cancers.

Breast cancer became the most common cancer globally as of 2021, accounting for 12% of all new annual cancer cases worldwide, according to the World Health Organization.

I will examine the Conventional Medicine (CM) explanations for breast cancer. You can reference these details in any mainstream conventional medicine website. They are all very similar with minor differences in detail. I will then contrast it with Dr. Ryke Geerd Hamer's explanation of the condition.

Dr. Hamer started his journey of understanding connections between the mind and body in 1978 when his 19-year-old son Dirk was shot and murdered. Two months after Dirk died, Dr. Hamer was diagnosed with testicular and stomach cancer. Receiving a cancer diagnosis of a reproductive organ two months after the untimely death of his 19-year-old son initiated a thought process in Dr. Hamer – surely the two were connected, but how?

The incident began Dr. Hamer's lifelong journey of discovery leading him to establish a new medical science, Germanic New Medicine (GNM) or Germanische Heilkunde (GHk). In English, this is loosely translated to Germanic Healing Knowledge.

I will share my personal experience of working with women with breast cancer. I will also make my own comments and observations on the different schools of thought.

I will assume that you have not heard of Dr. Ryke Geerd Hamer. It is a safe assumption, as most have not.

CHAPTER 1
BRIEF INTRODUCTION TO GERMANIC HEALING KNOWLEDGE (GHK)

The body of knowledge GHk or GNM is a form of mind-body medicine. Its founder, Dr. Ryke Geerd Hamer, was a traditionally-trained medical doctor from Germany. He specialized in internal medicine and medical research.

Every time we are faced with a challenge in life, our subconscious mind (or psyche as termed by Dr. Hamer), respond by increasing or decreasing our organ's capacity to help us solve that life challenge. This would be analogous to putting your foot on the accelerator or brake of your vehicle to avoid a road accident.

To increase our capacity, some parts of our body will add tissue when we face the problem, and remove tissue after we have solved it. In other parts of the body, it is the reverse. This process of adding and removing tissue leads to changes in the body's well-being and is generally what medical doctors call disease.

The easiest way to understand the process of tissue being added and removed is to look at a woman's menstrual cycle. In the first half of a woman's cycle, tissue is added to the walls of the uterus. If she does not get pregnant, the extra tissue is removed via bleeding, often accompanied by cramps and pain.

Dr. Hamer discovered that the testicular cancer he experienced after his son was murdered was not random and had a biological purpose. Increasing the functional tissue in the testicle increases testosterone and sperm production. This makes a man more fertile so he is better able to get a woman pregnant and replace the child he just lost.

According to Dr. Hamer, there are two types of breast cancer. A mammary gland cancer, and intraductal breast cancer. In the mammary gland cancer, tissue is added during the first phase called the conflict active phase, and removed when we resolve the conflict in the second, healing or repair phase. In intraductal breast cancer, it is the reverse. The milk ducts are ulcerated and widened during the conflict activity so tissue is removed, and restored during the healing or repair phase with inflammation and pain.

Dr. Hamer actually believed that there is only one form of breast cancer and that is mammary gland (lobular) cancer. Intraductal breast cancer is merely a replenishment process in the milk ducts.

Dr. Hamer believed that a replenishment process via inflammation and pain in the milk ducts is no more cancer than the inflammation and pain we experience when we cut our finger chopping vegetables in the kitchen. Read on to learn more about this.

If you want to test this medical science for yourself, think about something you really dislike, something in your life that really 'stinks' or 'sucks.' Think about it intensely. A little while after you start thinking about it, your nose will start running. A runny nose is caused by a 'stinking conflict.'

Now follow this exercise. Speak to your subconscious mind and say to it, "I know my nose is running because I was just thinking intensely about something I hate (fill in the blanks what you were just thinking about), please switch off my runny nose." What happened to your runny nose?

If there is a problem in your life that you have been 'biting your tongue' and not speaking about, gather the courage to talk about it. Soon after, your tongue will become hyper-sensitive, and you will get painful ulcers on the tongue!

Follow the same exercise with your tongue. Say to yourself, "I know my tongue is sore because I was biting my tongue about (fill in the blanks) and I gained the courage to speak about it."

Depending on how long you were biting your tongue on the issue, and how important the issue was to you, it will determine whether you either downgrade the pain on the tongue or switch it off completely. The longer you have bitten your tongue for, and the more important it was to you, the less the pain from the ulcers will reduce, and the longer they will take to heal.

Congratulations, you have just learned to switch biological programs (disease) on and off.

Once you have personal experience of how this medical science works, even deliberately making your nose run or tongue sore, it significantly increases your ability to believe that this medical science is the real deal. Every subsequent healing experience increases your conviction.

In my experience, it is the Holy Grail of health and wellness.

You can read a much more detailed explanation about Dr. Hamer and his medical discoveries in my book, **'Terminal Cancer is a Misdiagnosis.'**

CHAPTER 2
DANNY'S EXPERIENCE

Although men can suffer from breast cancer, I have not personally experienced it. However, I have worked with many women who have. I will share two case studies of women who came to me for help. One had a good outcome. Sadly, the other did not.

A right-handed lady in her 60s came to me after she had received a breast cancer diagnosis from a medical doctor. She had been for a mammogram and was diagnosed based on the results of the scan. She was not pleased with the diagnosis and was seeking second opinions.

I recommended she have a brain CT scan. Your entire life history is printed on your brain so every health issue can be diagnosed with one diagnostic test. The brain CT scan showed that she had suffered from breast cancer in the past, but it had fully resolved.

The mammogram showed areas of calcification in the breast. Medical doctors diagnose calcification as malignant cancer when it is in fact a fully resolved problem. When I explained to her that the problem was in the past and resolved long back, she said excitedly, "I knew there was no problem!" The lady decided not to go back to her doctor and got on with her life and put it down to a learning experience.

A right-handed woman in her 40s came to me after receiving a diagnosis of an aggressive intraductal breast cancer diagnosis on her right partner breast. She had regular fights with her husband, which caused the problem in the milk ducts in her right breast.

She had one foot in the conventional medicine camp and the other in the naturopathy camp, and oscillated between the two. Each time she hit a crisis point, she would come to me for help and then not come back for a long period. In between, she would go to the hospital for advice. This went on for a couple of years.

When the hospital did a biopsy, it made a small puncture close to her right nipple. The puncture did not heal and blood and pus continuously leaked from it. She was very proud of her breasts and this troubled her. She became obsessed with the blood leaking from the puncture and a melanoma started to develop around the puncture wound.

According to Dr. Hamer, melanoma is caused by an attack conflict and is nature's way of thickening the skin to help strengthen it against future attacks. In this case, the attack was caused by the puncture from the biopsy.

After the melanoma developed, doctors advised her to have a mastectomy and remove the breast. I strongly advised her against this. Due to her age, and her pride over her breasts, she had struggled to manage the consequences of a biopsy on the breast. If she agreed to the breast removal, my expectation was that the psychological impact on her could lead to dire consequences. And sadly, I was right.

She proceeded with the breast removal. This caused a huge problem for her and she said she no longer felt like a full woman and could not look at herself in the mirror. She was shocked by the look of her chest after the surgery and melanoma developed along the surgical scar.

Complications set in and she was subsequently diagnosed with pleural effusion. This is fluid between the chest cavity and the outside of the lung. According to Dr. Hamer, this is caused by an attack conflict on the chest. This would have been caused by the surgery to remove the breast.

The pleural effusion, combined with the prognosis (outlook) given by the hospital, triggered a fear of death or existence conflict. This triggered the survival function in her kidneys that causes water retention. This significantly increases the amount of fluid retained in the pleural cavity. This fluid is heavily concentrated with healing proteins.

She asked me if she should have a tap inserted to evacuate the fluid and I said it was not a good idea. Evacuating the healing fluids leads to excessive loss of protein in the body. So she followed the doctor's advice and had the tap inserted to evacuate the fluid from the pleural cavity.

Within two weeks of having the tap inserted, she died in her sleep. I foresaw this outcome long before it happened, but there was nothing I could do to prevent it.

The examples above show contrasting ways in which different people manage medical diagnoses, and the different outcomes that can result from the decisions made along the journey.

They also demonstrate the critical difference between what happens when you take responsibility for your own health versus outsourcing it to your medical doctor.

It always affects me deeply when somebody I have been trying to help passes away. Special bonds are developed in these situations. But I have to keep reminding myself that it is only possible to heal yourself. Some people can. Some people can't.

Dr. Hamer always used to say, it is difficult to teach someone to swim whilst they are in the process of drowning. It is always better to learn to swim before you enter the water.

Similarly, it is better to learn to heal yourself before you get sick. If you study Germanic Healing Knowledge and eliminate the fear of disease before you suffer health challenges, your chances of navigating them successfully increase dramatically, in my experience.

CHAPTER 3
CONVENTIONAL MEDICINE (CM) EXPLANATION FOR BREAST CANCER

Overview

Breast cancer is cancer that forms in the cells of the breasts.

After skin cancer, breast cancer is the most common cancer diagnosed in women in the United States. Breast cancer can occur in both men and women, but it's far more common in women.

Substantial support for breast cancer awareness and research funding has helped create advances in the diagnosis and treatment of breast cancer. Breast cancer survival rates have increased, and the number of deaths associated with this disease is steadily declining, largely due to factors such as earlier detection, a new personalized approach to treatment and a better understanding of the disease.

Types

Angiosarcoma

Angiosarcoma is a rare type of cancer that forms in the lining of the blood vessels and lymph vessels. The lymph vessels are part of the immune system. The lymph vessels collect bacteria, viruses and waste products from the body and dispose of them.

This type of cancer can occur any place in the body. But it most often occurs in the skin on the head and neck. Rarely, it may form in the skin on other parts of the body, such as the breast. Or it may form in deeper tissue, such as the liver and the heart. Angiosarcoma can occur in areas that were treated with radiation therapy in the past.

Treatment depends on where the cancer is located. Treatments may include surgery, radiation therapy and chemotherapy.

Ductal carcinoma in situ (DCIS)

Ductal carcinoma in situ (DCIS) is the presence of abnormal cells inside a milk duct in the breast.

DCIS is considered the earliest form of breast cancer. DCIS is non-invasive, meaning it hasn't spread out of the milk duct and has a low risk of becoming invasive.

DCIS is usually found during a mammogram done as part of breast cancer screening or to investigate a breast lump.

While DCIS isn't an emergency, it does require an evaluation and a consideration of treatment options. Treatment may include breast-conserving surgery combined with radiation or surgery to remove all of the breast tissue. A clinical trial studying active monitoring as an alternative to surgery may be another option.

Inflammatory breast cancer

Inflammatory breast cancer is a rare type of breast cancer that develops rapidly, making the affected breast red, swollen and tender.

Inflammatory breast cancer occurs when cancer cells block the lymphatic vessels in skin covering the breast, causing the characteristic red, swollen appearance of the breast.

Inflammatory breast cancer is considered a locally advanced cancer meaning it has spread from its point of origin to nearby tissue and possibly to nearby lymph nodes.

Inflammatory breast cancer can easily be confused with a breast infection, which is a much more common cause of breast redness and swelling. Seek medical attention promptly if you notice skin changes on your breast.

Invasive lobular carcinoma

Invasive lobular carcinoma is a type of breast cancer that begins in the milk-producing glands (lobules) of the breast.

Invasive cancer means the cancer cells have broken out of the lobule where they began and have the potential to spread to the lymph nodes and other areas of the body.

Invasive lobular carcinoma makes up a small portion of all breast cancers. The most common type of breast cancer begins in the breast ducts (invasive ductal carcinoma).

Lobular carcinoma in situ (LCIS)

Lobular carcinoma in situ (LCIS) is an uncommon condition in which abnormal cells form in the milk glands (lobules) in the breast. LCIS isn't cancer. But being diagnosed with LCIS indicates that you have an increased risk of developing breast cancer.

LCIS usually doesn't show up on mammograms. The condition is most often discovered as a result of a breast biopsy done for another reason, such as a suspicious breast lump or an abnormal mammogram.

Women with LCIS have an increased risk of developing invasive breast cancer in either breast. If you're diagnosed with LCIS, your doctor may recommend increased breast cancer screening and may ask you to consider medical treatments to reduce your risk of developing invasive breast cancer.

Male breast cancer

Male breast cancer is a rare cancer that forms in the breast tissue of men. Though breast cancer is most commonly thought of as a disease that affects women, breast cancer does occur in men.

Male breast cancer is most common in older men, though it can occur at any age.

Men diagnosed with male breast cancer at an early stage have a good chance for a cure. Treatment typically involves surgery to remove the breast tissue. Other treatments, such as chemotherapy and radiation therapy, may be recommended based on your particular situation.

Paget's disease of the breast

Paget's (PAJ-its) disease of the breast is a rare form of breast cancer. Paget's disease of the breast starts on the nipple and extends to the dark circle of skin (areola) around the nipple. Paget's disease of the breast isn't related to Paget's disease of the bone, a metabolic bone disease.

Paget's disease of the breast occurs most often after age 50. Most people with this diagnosis also have underlying ductal breast cancer, either in situ — meaning in its original place — or, less commonly, invasive breast cancer. Only rarely is Paget's disease of the breast confined to the nipple itself.

Recurrent breast cancer

Recurrent breast cancer is breast cancer that comes back after initial treatment. Although the initial treatment is aimed at eliminating all cancer cells, a few may have evaded treatment and survived. These undetected cancer cells multiply, becoming recurrent breast cancer.

Recurrent breast cancer may occur months or years after your initial treatment. The cancer may come back in the same place as the original cancer (local recurrence), or it may spread to other areas of your body (distant recurrence).

Learning you have recurrent breast cancer may be harder than dealing with the initial diagnosis. But having recurrent breast cancer is far from hopeless. Treatment may eliminate local, regional or distant recurrent breast cancer. Even if a cure isn't possible, treatment may control the disease for long periods of time.

Symptoms

Signs and symptoms of breast cancer may include:

- A breast lump or thickening that feels different from the surrounding tissue
- Change in the size, shape or appearance of a breast
- Changes to the skin over the breast, such as dimpling
- A newly inverted nipple
- Peeling, scaling, crusting or flaking of the pigmented area of skin surrounding the nipple (areola) or breast skin

- Redness or pitting of the skin over your breast, like the skin of an orange

When to see a doctor

If you find a lump or other change in your breast — even if a recent mammogram was normal — make an appointment with your doctor for prompt evaluation.

Causes

Doctors know that breast cancer occurs when some breast cells begin to grow abnormally. These cells divide more rapidly than healthy cells do and continue to accumulate, forming a lump or mass. Cells may spread (metastasize) through your breast to your lymph nodes or to other parts of your body.

Breast cancer most often begins with cells in the milk-producing ducts (invasive ductal carcinoma). Breast cancer may also begin in the glandular tissue called lobules (invasive lobular carcinoma) or in other cells or tissue within the breast.

Researchers have identified hormonal, lifestyle and environmental factors that may increase your risk of breast cancer. But it's not clear why some people who have no risk factors develop cancer, yet other people with risk factors never do. It's likely that breast cancer is caused by a complex interaction of your genetic makeup and your environment.

Inherited breast cancer

Doctors estimate that about 5 to 10 percent of breast cancers are linked to gene mutations passed through generations of a family.

A number of inherited mutated genes that can increase the likelihood of breast cancer have been identified. The most well-known are breast cancer gene 1 (BRCA1) and breast cancer gene 2 (BRCA2), both of which significantly increase the risk of both breast and ovarian cancer.

If you have a strong family history of breast cancer or other cancers, your doctor may recommend a blood test to help identify specific mutations in BRCA or other genes that are being passed through your family.

Consider asking your doctor for a referral to a genetic counselor, who can review your family health history. A genetic counselor can also discuss the benefits, risks and limitations of genetic testing to assist you with shared decision-making.

Risk factors

A breast cancer risk factor is anything that makes it more likely you'll get breast cancer. But having one or even several breast cancer risk factors doesn't necessarily mean you'll develop breast cancer. Many women who develop breast cancer have no known risk factors other than simply being women.

Factors that are associated with an increased risk of breast cancer include:

- **Being female.** Women are much more likely than men are to develop breast cancer.
- **Increasing age.** Your risk of breast cancer increases as you age.
- **A personal history of breast conditions.** If you've had a breast biopsy that found lobular carcinoma in situ (LCIS) or atypical hyperplasia of the breast, you have an increased risk of breast cancer.
- **A personal history of breast cancer.** If you've had breast cancer in one breast, you have an increased risk of developing cancer in the other breast.
- **A family history of breast cancer.** If your mother, sister or daughter was diagnosed with

breast cancer, particularly at a young age, your risk of breast cancer is increased. Still, the majority of people diagnosed with breast cancer have no family history of the disease.

- **Inherited genes that increase cancer risk.** Certain gene mutations that increase the risk of breast cancer can be passed from parents to children. The most well-known gene mutations are referred to as BRCA1 and BRCA2. These genes can greatly increase your risk of breast cancer and other cancers, but they don't make cancer inevitable.
- **Radiation exposure.** If you received radiation treatments to your chest as a child or young adult, your risk of breast cancer is increased.
- **Obesity.** Being obese increases your risk of breast cancer.
- **Beginning your period at a younger age.** Beginning your period before age 12 increases your risk of breast cancer.
- **Beginning menopause at an older age.** If you began menopause at an older age, you're more likely to develop breast cancer.
- **Having your first child at an older age.** Women who give birth to their first child after age 30 may have an increased risk of breast cancer.

- **Having never been pregnant.** Women who have never been pregnant have a greater risk of breast cancer than do women who have had one or more pregnancies.
- **Postmenopausal hormone therapy.** Women who take hormone therapy medications that combine estrogen and progesterone to treat the signs and symptoms of menopause have an increased risk of breast cancer. The risk of breast cancer decreases when women stop taking these medications.
- **Drinking alcohol.** Drinking alcohol increases the risk of breast cancer.

Prevention

Breast cancer risk reduction for women with an average risk

Making changes in your daily life may help reduce your risk of breast cancer. Try to:

- **Ask your doctor about breast cancer screening.** Discuss with your doctor when to begin breast cancer screening exams and tests, such as clinical breast exams and mammograms.

Talk to your doctor about the benefits and risks of screening. Together, you can decide what breast cancer screening strategies are right for you.

- **Become familiar with your breasts through breast self-exam for breast awareness.** Women may choose to become familiar with their breasts by occasionally inspecting their breasts during a breast self-exam for breast awareness. If there is a new change, lumps or other unusual signs in your breasts, talk to your doctor promptly.

Breast awareness can't prevent breast cancer, but it may help you to better understand the normal changes that your breasts undergo and identify any unusual signs and symptoms.

- **Drink alcohol in moderation, if at all.** Limit the amount of alcohol you drink to no more than one drink a day, if you choose to drink.
- **Exercise most days of the week.** Aim for at least 30 minutes of exercise on most days of the week. If you haven't been active lately, ask your doctor whether it's OK and start slowly.
- **Limit postmenopausal hormone therapy.** Combination hormone therapy may increase

the risk of breast cancer. Talk with your doctor about the benefits and risks of hormone therapy.

Some women experience bothersome signs and symptoms during menopause and, for these women, the increased risk of breast cancer may be acceptable in order to relieve menopause signs and symptoms.

To reduce the risk of breast cancer, use the lowest dose of hormone therapy possible for the shortest amount of time.

- **Maintain a healthy weight.** If your weight is healthy, work to maintain that weight. If you need to lose weight, ask your doctor about healthy strategies to accomplish this. Reduce the number of calories you eat each day and slowly increase the amount of exercise.
- **Choose a healthy diet.** Women who eat a Mediterranean diet supplemented with extra-virgin olive oil and mixed nuts may have a reduced risk of breast cancer. The Mediterranean diet focuses mostly on plant-based foods, such as fruits and vegetables, whole grains, legumes, and nuts. People who

follow the Mediterranean diet choose healthy fats, such as olive oil, over butter and fish instead of red meat.

Breast cancer risk reduction for women with a high risk

If your doctor has assessed your family history and determined that you have other factors, such as a precancerous breast condition, that increase your risk of breast cancer, you may discuss options to reduce your risk, such as:

- **Preventive medications (chemoprevention).** Estrogen-blocking medications, such as selective estrogen receptor modulators and aromatase inhibitors, reduce the risk of breast cancer in women with a high risk of the disease.

These medications carry a risk of side effects, so doctors reserve these medications for women who have a very high risk of breast cancer. Discuss the benefits and risks with your doctor.

- **Preventive surgery.** Women with a very high risk of breast cancer may choose to have their healthy breasts surgically removed (prophylactic mastectomy). They may also choose to have their healthy ovaries removed (prophylactic oophorectomy) to reduce the risk of both breast cancer and ovarian cancer.

CHAPTER 4
DR. HAMER'S EXPLANATION OF BREAST CANCER

The description of Dr. Hamer's explanation for breast cancer and case studies is taken from Dr. Hamer's Scientific Chart (**https://amici-di-dirk.com**), Helmut Pilhar's seminar on breast cancer, Bjorn Eybl's book The Psychic Roots of Disease (**https://free-new-medicine.com**), and Dr. Caroline Markolin's website (**https://learninggnm.com**).

According to Germanic Healing Knowledge, there are only two forms of breast cancer. The most common is intraductal breast cancer, which affects the milk ducts in the breast. The second is mammary gland (lobular) cancer. This, as the name describes, affects the mammary glands in the breast.

As mentioned in the introduction, Dr. Hamer believed that intraductal breast cancer is a cell replenishment process similar to when your finger heals when you cut it and is not 'abnormal cell multiplication' as cancer is defined by conventional medicine and should never have been classified as cancer. But it has.

In Germanic Healing Knowledge, nature's biological programs work in two phases. This is Dr. Hamer's second biological law, "The Law of Two Phases."

All diseases, or 'biological programs' as Dr. Hamer called them, go through these two phases. The first phase is the "conflict active" phase. The second phase, post resolving the conflict, is called the "healing or repair" phase.

In mammary gland cancer, tissue is added during the first, conflict-active phase, and removed during the second, healing and repair phase.

For intraductal cancer, it is the reverse. Tissue is removed during conflict activity, and replenished during the healing or repair phase.

Handedness

Determining whether a person is left or right brain-wired is critically important when diagnosing the conflict that triggered the problem to start in relation to the mammary gland and intraductal cancer.

If you are right-handed, or right-brain-wired, if your left breast is affected by cancer, the problem is triggered by a conflict with your mother or child. The right breast is affected by a conflict with everybody else. If you are left brain-wired, it is the reverse.

Just because you write with your right hand does not always mean you are right brain-wired. My wife writes with her right hand but is left brain-wired.

Some religious groups believe that left-handed people are evil. They force young left-handed children to write with their right hand. They are known to follow practices like tying children's left hand behind their backs to force them to write with their right hand.

Determining which way your brain is wired is a critical step to ensuring you are looking for the conflict in the correct relationship that caused the problem to start. ***And finding the initial conflict that triggered the conflict is the key to solving the problem.***

There are a number of tests you can use to determine your brain-wiring and true laterality.

The clap test

Try clapping your hands. Your dominant hand is normally on top. If you are right-handed, your right hand will be on top and your left hand below. If you are left-handed, it is the reverse. If you clap like patty cake with both hands parallel in front of you, try the next test.

The nail file test

Try filing your fingernails. You will typically use your dominant hand to file your nails. If you are right brain-wired, whilst filing the nails on your right hand, you will hold the file in your left hand but the movement to file the nails will come from your right hand. It is the reverse for people who are left brain-wired.

Carry a baby test

Try carrying a baby, or a doll to simulate a baby. If you are right brain-wired, you will rest the baby's head on your left shoulder and support the baby's weight with your dominant right arm under the baby's bottom. If you are left-handed, it is the reverse.

The swirl of the crown of your hair test

If you check the crown of your hair at the top of your head, it will have a swirl. The swirl can go clockwise or anti-clockwise. If the swirl is clockwise, it means you are right brain-wired. If it is anti-clockwise, it means you are left brain-wired.

This test is much easier to do with people who have short hair as it is easier to see the swirl in the crown. If you have long hair, wait until your hair is wet after you have washed it, and then open up the hair and check the crown for the swirl.

Case Study Examples

Mammary Gland Cancer

*A 43-year-old, left-handed woman is blamed by her daughter for having destroyed her marriage. This is a mother-child fight conflict. A tumor of the right mother-child breast develops. (Archive, B. Eybl)

*A right-handed woman embarks on a week-long vacation with friends, while her ex-husband cares for their epileptic daughter. On the very first day of the vacation, she receives a phone call from home. Her ex-husband reports that their daughter has had a severe epileptic fit and is currently in the hospital. He blames his ex-wife (the patient) for not being there.

She wants to fly back to her daughter right away but is unable to book a flight. This is a mother-child worry conflict. She experienced one week of very strong conflict activity. A breast-gland tumor develops in the left breast. In the following years, the patient remains mildly conflict active because she is expecting another fit at any time.

Not until the daughter has been stable for several years does she come into healing. The patient sweats at night, the breast reddens, swells up and after six weeks breaks open and gives off stinking pus. (Archive, B. Eybl)

*A woman moves to a large city in a colder climate for her education where she has to accept living in a dark, inner-courtyard apartment. Accustomed to a sunny climate, she is unhappy in the apartment and longs for life-giving sunlight.

She comes to the conclusion that "everything is so dark in this land." This caused a nest conflict. To relieve her distress, she moves her bed right up to the window so she can 'catch' a little light. Subsequently, she is diagnosed with breast gland cancer. (Archive, Antje Scherret)

*40-year-old right-handed man. His wife cheated on him regularly. He got a lump in his left chest as his wife was too busy with other men and not looking after their children. He left her and remarried. He had a child with his second wife who was a good mother.

Having a good mother for his children resolved his conflict. In the healing phase, the surface skin broke and he had a large open wound on his chest that smelled very bad and festered. This lasted for many months, during which time he thought it was just an abscess.

15 years later, the man went to Dr. Hamer. When he read his brain CT scan, Dr. Hamer informed that man that he previously had breast cancer. (Archive, Helmut Pilhar)

*27-year-old right-handed woman. Her one-year-old child was screaming in the kitchen. The child put both hands on the electric stove and got badly burned. The mother rushed the child to the hospital and stayed in the hospital with the child.

After a few days, she felt a lump in her left breast. Seeing that she was still breastfeeding, she thought nothing of it. She lay in bed in the hospital at night and couldn't sleep as she was constantly thinking about her child's injuries.

She had previously been told about GHk so spent her time in the hospital researching breast cancer case studies in GHk. She read case studies that were very similar to the situation she was in. Her mouth fell open when she read the case studies. Due to the knowledge she had acquired during the hospital stay, she was able to resolve the conflict at the end of the first hospitalization and the lump soon disappeared. (Archive, Helmut Pilhar)

*Right-handed woman 17-year-old fell in love with her horse riding teacher. The teacher wanted to end the untenable relationship. The woman went into a mental constellation and went crazy.

She went to Dr. Hamer and when he looked at her brain CT, she had also responded with breast cancer that she had not noticed. Dr. Hamer predicted that she would soon feel a lump in her breast.

A few weeks later, she could feel the lump in her breast. She had a diagnosis in CM who diagnosed it as malignant. Because she already knew about the lump and what caused it, she ignored the medical diagnosis.

The mammary gland tissue added during conflict activity is normally removed naturally by tuberculosis mycobacteria. If you have had frequent doses of antibiotics as a child, this tuberculosis mycobacteria is killed in the body and the extra tissue cannot be removed and the extra tissue becomes an encapsulated cyst.

She had no mycobacteria to remove the lump so it became encapsulated. At the age of 35, the lump still remained. She said it did not bother her, it was now just a part of her.

*Right-handed 50-year-old woman. Had a lump in her breast on her mother-child side. She went to the hospital and had a biopsy and was diagnosed with malignant breast cancer.

She asked the doctor the cause and he said it was caused by environmental toxins, heredity, stress, smoking, etc. The doctors' prognosis (outlook) was, that if she didn't go immediately for surgery, she would not survive for 4 weeks.

The lady discovered GHk before the surgery. After establishing her correct laterality, the GHk consultant asked about her life regarding her mother and children.

The lady had a 29-year-old son from a previous marriage who drank himself to death. She found him in bed dead one morning. This was a terrible unexpected shock for the lady.

She spent the next 6 months with the GHk consultant working through the healing symptoms and at the end of that period, the lump shrank and ended up as a tiny encapsulated lump in her breast. (Archive, Helmut Pilhar)

*30-year-old right-handed woman. The physician assistant takes mammograms all day long. She notices a 4cm lump in her breast. Knowing the treatment she will get in conventional medicine, she went to a natural healer.

She was referred to Dr. Hamer. Dr Hamer diagnosed a conflict in her mother-child breast. This was caused by a worry over her mother who had received a colon cancer diagnosis.

The woman was wise and made a commitment that if her mother was diagnosed with cancer again, she would not let her go to CM again and she would help her mother.

With this, she resolved her care conflict and came into healing. During the healing, she experienced an epileptic fit, which means she also had experienced a motor conflict. She had not noticed the partial paralysis in the conflict-active phase.

6 months later, she got pregnant and gave birth to a healthy child and breast feed the child from the breast where she had mammary gland cancer. (Archive, Helmut Pilhar)

Intraductal Breast Cancer

*A left-handed, happily married woman has a son, whom she loves above all else. At the beginning of his studies, he is still living at home with his parents. She is severely affected by his announcement that he plans to move into his own apartment. She never imagined that he would leave so quickly. For her, he was always her 'little boy.'

This is a conflict of her son is being pulled away from her breast. This caused an unnoticed cell degradation in the milk ducts in the active phase.

One day, after the patient accepted that her son's leaving is a positive and normal development, she notices a lump in her right mother-child breast. CM: invasive ductal carcinoma. (Archive Claudio Trupiano, thanks to Dr. Hamer)

*A 39-year-old, right-handed woman has a number of fierce disagreements with her husband about his ex-wife. In her opinion, he is too friendly and cooperative toward her.

This caused a partner-separation conflict affecting the milk ducts of the right breast. This caused an unnoticed cell loss in the active phase, and restoration of the milk ducts (intraductal cancer) in the repair phase. (Archive, B. Eybl)

*A 41-year-old, childless, right-handed patient has a dog named Benni whom she loves very much. She makes it clear to her mother, who lives on a farm, that she mustn't lay out any rat poison because that could endanger Benni. Her mother ignores her warnings and misfortune strikes: Benni eats the poison and dies.

Her pet child is 'pulled away from the breast.' She doesn't want to talk about it to anyone, because Benni was "just a dog." This caused cell loss in the active phase.

Not until a year later, does the patient recover from the incident. In the repair phase, she notices a white lesion on the left nipple. A 2x2x4 cm lump develops in the milk ducts. The patient is relieved as she learns about the causal relationships and refuses CM treatment. Within a year, the lump is almost gone. (Archive, B. Eybl)

*A 42-year-old, right-handed married patient, mother of two children, has a husband who is very much under his mother's influence. The patient's mother-in-law tries to pull the two children onto her side and this has nearly ruined their marriage.

One Christmas, her husband takes the children 'for a quick visit' to his parents. However, he and the children stay and celebrate with the mother-in-law. This caused a mother-child separation conflict. The children are "torn from her breast." (Archive, B. Eybl)

*10-year-old right-handed boy. A young boy loved snow-boarding. His class went on a ski course and they could choose between skiing and snowboarding. The class choose skiing. The boy became stubborn and said he would not go skiing so had to go back to class on his own his.

His nipple on his partner's side became retracted as he had a separation conflict from his class. When the class returned, it started healing and became very painful. (Archive, Helmut Pilhar)

Conflict (The cause of the problem)

Mammary Gland Cancer

Mammary gland cancer is caused by what Dr. Hamer described as a "nest worry or care" conflict. During the evolutionary development process, the breast was a key tool available to a woman to nurse a sick loved one back to health.

When a woman (or man if he has low testosterone levels), experiences a "nest worry or care" conflict, nature re-activates the mammary glands in the breast so that the mother can restart lactation and offer her breast to the sick loved one to help nurse them back to full health.

Intraductal Breast Cancer

In Germanic Healing Knowledge, intraductal breast cancer is caused by a "separation conflict." It is a conflict of someone being "torn away from my breast." If you are right-brain-wired, the left breast gets affected by separation conflicts with your mother or children. Your right breast gets affected by separation conflicts with everyone else. If you are left-brain-wired, it is the reverse.

A pet that you treat like a child will affect the left breast of a right-handed woman. An elderly father whom you look after like a child can also affect the mother-child left breast. It is dependent on the nature of your relationship.

The separation conflict can be both someone whom you are separated from and want to be reunited with, or a wanted separation that you cannot achieve i.e. someone you are with whom you want to be separated from.

Conflict Activity (When the problem starts)

In both intraductal and mammary cancer, the biological program (or disease) is triggered in the very instant of experiencing the separation conflict in intraductal breast cancer, and the nest worry or care conflict in mammary gland cancer. In a split second, the shock affects the psyche, brain, and organ, like an electric shock.

Dr. Hamer named this unexpected biological conflict shock in memory of his son Dirk. In Germanic Healing Knowledge, the unexpected conflict shock is called Dirk Hamer Syndrome, or DHS.

There are three criteria for this conflict shock to trigger a "cancer" program. The shock has to be unexpected, highly acute, and isolative. Dr. Hamer described this as being "caught on the wrong foot." This puts you in a high state of stress and you think about the problem continuously until you resolve the conflict.

Nature will wake you up at 3:00 am to give you more waking hours to solve the problem. Your extremities, hands and feet, will become cold due to reduced blood circulation. You will also have very little appetite and will lose weight.

In mammary gland cancer, the tumor starts growing as soon as you experience nest worry or care conflict.

In intraductal cancer, there is no pain when you experience the separation conflict shock, the milk ducts ulcerate and widen. If the conflict lasts for a long time, the nipple and surrounding areola become numb.

If the separation conflict is either long-running, intense, or re-occurring conflicts, it can lead to knots developing in the milk ducts. This is diagnosed by CM as a scirrhous carcinoma.

According to Dr. Hamer, this is not cancer at all. It is just scar tissue. No different to when you cut your finger multiple times cutting vegetables. After you have cut it multiple times, scar tissue builds up. If scar tissue builds up in the milk ducts and they become shorter in length, the nipple can also become inverted.

The scar tissue is designed to strengthen the skin to protect it and make it stronger if it gets cut again in the future.

How would you react if the medical doctor diagnosed the scar on your finger as a scirrhous carcinoma? Would you let him chop off your finger? The same principle applies to the milk ducts and the breast.

You will also experience short-term memory loss.

Biological Purpose or Meaning

One of Dr. Hamer's many extraordinary medical discoveries was that all biological changes that happen in the human body have a biological purpose or meaning. Evolution has developed human biology to maximize our chances of survival. An increase or decrease in an organ system's capacity can help us in times of trouble to survive difficult challenges in life.

Mammary Gland Cancer

With mammary gland cancer, the biological purpose or meaning is in the first conflict-active phase and is to reactivate the mammary gland's capacity to produce milk so that you can offer your breast to a sick loved one to nurse them back to full health.

Unfortunately, the understanding of the importance of the breast as a nurturing tool has been largely lost in today's society.

Intraductal Breast Cancer

With intraductal cancer, the biological purpose or meaning is also in the first conflict-active phase. In nature's design, when a mother is separated from her child, the milk is no longer being suckled from the breast and needs to be evacuated.

In the conflict-active phase, the milk ducts ulcerate and widen so that the unconsumed milk can more easily be drained from the breast. Again, in today's modern society, the biological purpose of this program can be difficult for us to relate to.

The nipple also becomes numb. The biological purpose of this is to help you forget about the physical contact you are missing with your breast. This is accompanied by short-term memory loss. This is also nature's design to help you forget about the person you are separated from.

Conflict Resolution or Repair Phase (After the problem has been resolved)

Mammary Gland Cancer

In mammary gland cancer, conflict resolution means that your nest worry or care conflict has been resolved. If a loved one in your nest was sick, they have now recovered their health and you no longer need the capacity to offer them your breast.

Mammary gland tissue is added in the first conflict-active phase and removed in the repair or healing phase. This added tissue (or tumor) is removed with fungi and tuberculosis mycobacteria. Healing symptoms include swelling and sharp pain.

Whenever a healing program involving tuberculosis mycobacteria is running, you will experience night sweats. When you wake up in the morning, your bed sheets will be soaking wet. You will also have zero energy. You will need to sleep or rest for large parts of the day.

If you have had heavy doses of antibiotics that have killed your natural tuberculosis mycobacteria, the tumor cannot be removed. It will develop into a cyst and remain in the breast as a hard lump.

If the tuberculosis mycobacteria break the surface skin of the breast, blood and foul-smelling discharge will come out of the open wound. This smells like rotting flesh. Which is exactly what it is. The tuberculosis mycobacteria remove the tissue added during conflict activity by rotting the tissue. If the outer layer of skin breaks, the smell is putrid and very unpleasant.

If the breast breaks open, protein-rich healing fluids will leak from the open wound in the breast. It is critical that these proteins are replaced through a protein-heavy diet. It is not recommended that you experiment with raw food or low-protein vegetarian diets at this point.

If you experience weight loss during this period, if you do not increase your protein intake, it can lead to cachexia, which is a wasting away of muscle and fats in the body. If you do not replace the lost proteins through your diet, nature will steal them from your muscles. Nature prioritizes applying the proteins from your muscles to the healing process.

The time that it takes to heal depends on the length of time you were in conflict and the amount of added tissue that has built up, multiplied by the intensity of the conflict. The longer the conflict has run and the more intense the conflict, the longer it will take to heal.

Intraductal Breast Cancer

In intraductal cancer, the tissue is removed from the milk duct in the conflict-active phase. In the healing or repair phase, the milk ducts are repaired with inflammation, pain, and itching. The nipple can again become inverted during the healing process. When the milk ducts swell up, milk ducts become shorter in length and temporarily pull the nipple inside the breast.

In nature's design, once the separation conflict has been resolved, the infant would normally resume suckling from the breast. Although milk is not being produced, the healing fluids in the breast make the breast swollen and engorged. The ducts become blocked with inflammation and the healing fluids cannot drain off.

If the healing fluids are not drained from the breast, the breast will shrink and it will become small and hard once the healing process has been completed. This can be prevented if the fluid is evacuated from the breast. This can either be done with a breast pump, or a partner can suckle the breast and remove it.

Animals suffer from the same biological conflicts as humans. When a calf is taken away from a cow, the cow also suffers from a separation conflict. The cow will resolve this conflict when she has another calf. One of the cow's udders will become inflamed and painful. Farmers call this quarter pain.

To help it heal, the farmer will milk the udder only by hand, not by a machine. When the udder is milked by hand, it evacuates the milk in the udder and helps the milk ducts to clear any blockage. If you consult any farmer, he will explain how the udder heals in a short period of time after milking.

Dr. Hamer had a practical tip he always advised his patients: The inflammation on the breast can be relieved by applying crushed leaves of a savoy cabbage on the inflamed breast. Remove the thick ribs from the leaves and insert the leaf inside your bra. This helps to soften the breast and reduce inflammation. You can also apply milking grease to the inflamed breast. This will help the skin on the breast from becoming dry and brittle.

Inflammation and pain are almost always a sign of healing. The biological purpose of pain is to stop you from using a part of the body so that it has the time, space and energy required to heal. When you cut your finger, it swells up and becomes painful. The pain is there to stop you from using it.

At the end of the healing process, it becomes intensely itchy. The healing process of the milk ducts in the breast follows exactly the same healing process.

If you have any form of calcification in the breast, this is also formed after the conflict has been fully resolved. CM will often diagnose calcification as malignant breast cancer. This is a misdiagnosis.

Healing Crisis (Nature's way of removing inflammation from the brain and organ after healing is completed)

Healing can only happen in a fluid environment. Once the healing process is complete, the body needs to remove the healing fluid from both the organ and the brain relay that manages this organ. This Dr. Hamer named the healing crisis. The inflammation is squeezed out of the organ and the brain.

The body achieves this by temporarily putting you back into conflict activity. You will re-experience the nest worry or separation conflict emotions that triggered the conflict and the biological program to start. This can last from seconds to weeks, depending on how much fluid has built up in the brain and organ.

In mammary gland cancer, this will involve chills or feeling cold, coupled with severe pain.

In intraductal cancer, you also experience short-term memory loss again. This can range from a conscious absence where you just feel spaced out, to fainting and losing consciousness. If you do faint, it is important to tell people close to you not to attempt to wake you up.

If the body needs to remove healing fluid from your brain, sometimes it has to shut systems down to remove it. That means making you unconscious. If you disturb this process and fluid is not removed from the brain, it will keep happening until the fluid is removed.

Your blood sugar levels will drop during the healing crisis. The brain uses a lot of glucose during the healing crisis. It is important to eat or drink something with high sugar levels after you have experienced short-term memory loss, especially if you fainted and fell unconscious.

CHAPTER 5
DANNY'S COMMENTS AND OBSERVATIONS

Cause

The most obvious difference between Conventional Medicine (CM) and Germanic Healing Knowledge (GHk) lies in the understanding of the cause of breast cancer.

According to CM:

"Researchers have identified hormonal, lifestyle and environmental factors that may increase your risk of breast cancer. But it's not clear why some people who have no risk factors develop cancer, yet other people with risk factors never do. It's likely that breast cancer is caused by a complex interaction of your genetic makeup and your environment."

"Doctors estimate that about 5 to 10 percent of breast cancers are linked to gene mutations passed through generations of a family.

A number of inherited mutated genes that can increase the likelihood of breast cancer have been identified. The most well-known are breast cancer gene 1 (BRCA1) and breast cancer gene 2 (BRCA2), both of which significantly increase the risk of both breast and ovarian cancer."

"A breast cancer risk factor is anything that makes it more likely you'll get breast cancer. But having one or even several breast cancer risk factors doesn't necessarily mean you'll develop breast cancer. Many women who develop breast cancer have no known risk factors other than simply being women."

This is my favourite:

***A family history of breast cancer.** If your mother, sister or daughter was diagnosed with breast cancer, particularly at a young age, your risk of breast cancer is increased. Still, the majority of people diagnosed with breast cancer have no family history of the disease.*

Is your understanding of the risks of breast cancer clearer now?

In GHk, breast cancer is caused by experiencing a nest worry or care conflict in the case of mammary gland cancer. In intraductal cancer, it is caused by a separation conflict with a loved one. This is either being separated from someone you want to be with or wanting to separate from someone you are with.

CM description of what they believe the cause to be is far from convincing. Apparently, you can have all the risk factors and never get breast cancer, or have none of them and get breast cancer. And the first listed risk factor is if you are a woman. And if you have a close family member who has had breast cancer, your risk increases. But the majority of women diagnosed have no family history.

You can follow all prevention recommendations, follow a Mediterranean diet, not drink alcohol, exercise regularly, maintain good body weight, and brush your teeth twice a day, but it appears if you are a woman, your risk profile will remain the same.

If you are considered to be a high risk, you can always consider having your healthy breasts removed, as Angelina Jolie did. What the doctors do not explain is that even if the breasts have been removed, you can still get breast cancer. This is described by CM as recurrent breast cancer. The biological program for breast cancer runs in your brain and not the organ, so it makes no difference if the organ is still there or not.

A good example of how removing an organ does not solve a problem is shown by what doctors calls 'phantom limb pain.' Phantom limb pain is where amputees still experience pain in a limb after the limb has been amputated. The Cleveland Clinic[I] reports that eight out of ten people who have limbs amputated still experience pain in the limb despite its absence.

This begs the question: How does someone feel pain in a limb that is no longer there? This is like having a fire in your barn after it was removed from your property. Absurd, right?

So, what is the explanation for phantom limb pain? The answer is: The pain is in the brain, not the limb/organ. It doesn't matter whether the organ is still there or not. The biological program, which is resulting in pain, is still running in the brain.

All biological programs, or diseases, as the doctors call them (except for poisoning, injuries from accidents, and nutritional deficiency diseases, e.g., scurvy through a lack of vitamin C), are caused by our psyche's perception of unexpected, distressing, external events. The brain is the control center where the program runs, and the organ expresses the program.

You can never solve the problem at the organ level. The organ expresses the symptoms of the program, it is not the cause.

Recurrent breast cancer on a breast that has been removed, and phantom limb pain are good examples that clearly demonstrates this.

Having a breast removed has little or no effect on the risk of getting breast cancer. If you want to eliminate your risk of breast cancer by removing organs, it appears the only viable option would be to have your head amputated. And this is far from an ideal solution.

Biological Purpose

Mammary Gland Cancer

According to Dr. Hamer, cancer is not a disease. It is a biological program that has a biological purpose or meaning. The female breast is a nurturing piece of biological equipment. Outside of the period of child-birth and breastfeeding, a woman does not lactate and produce milk.

Nature has designed our biology to maximize our chances of survival. For the breast, this means in times of trouble, re-activating a woman's ability to lactate outside the period of childbirth and breastfeeding. This gives a woman the ability to nurse a sick loved one back to health regardless of their age.

The mammary glands in the breast is triggered to re-activate milk production by a nest worry or care conflict. If you are walking down the road talking to a friend and not paying attention and your 5-year-old pulls away from you and runs in the road, gets hit by a car and ends up in the hospital, it will trigger the activation of the mammary gland in your mother-child breast.

The biological purpose is for the breast to restart producing milk so you can nurse your child back to health. I find this biological program easier to understand than most as it just makes sense. It is a gift from nature. This is what CM calls a lobular carcinoma.

Intraductal Breast Cancer

The biological program of the milk ducts can be more difficult to understand. Imagine a sheep nursing a lamb. A fox comes and takes the lamb away. The sheep now has an udder full of milk and no lamb to suckle it dry. The milk, therefore, has to be evacuated otherwise the udder will reach bursting point.

With intraductal breast cancer, when you experience the separation conflict, it is biologically the equivalent of the lamb being taken from the sheep, that is "somebody was torn from my breast." The milk ducts ulcerate and widen during the first conflict-active phase.

The biological purpose is so the milk ducts become wider for the milk to better be evacuated. This is more difficult to understand when you are not pregnant and do not have milk in your breast to evacuate. It took me a bit more time to get my head around this biological meaning.

The nipple becoming numb and short-term memory loss are also part of the biological purpose of this biological program. This is nature's way of helping you to forget about the person you are missing, and to make the nipple numb to help forget about the physical contact. This part of the biological program, I find, is easier to understand as it again, just makes logical sense.

Metastasis

According to modern medicine, cancer cells break off tumors and swim through your bloodstream or lymphatic system and attack other organs. What we are not told is, that this is just a hypothesis. A cancer cell, malignant or benign, has never been found in either the bloodstream or lymphatic systems.

If there were really cancer cells swimming around your bloodstream, would your blood not have to be screened for cancer cells when you donate it?

The most common secondary or metastatic cancers are of the lung, liver and lymph glands. Isn't it strange that breast cancer only generally affects one breast and cancer does not metastasize to the second breast when it is made from the same tissue and lives right next door?

According to NIH (National Institute of Health) in a cancer research study titled published in 2019 "National Trends of Bilateral Breast Cancer Incidence in the United States,"[1] "the incidence of bilateral breast cancer (cancer in both breasts) increased significantly from 1.4% in 1975 to 2.9% in 2014."

Even though the incidence of Bilateral breast cancer has more than doubled since 1975, in more than 97% of breast cancer cases, cancer does not metastasize to the second breast.

The main tissue in the lung is called the alveoli. According to Dr. Hamer, it is affected by a fear of death or existence conflict for self or a loved one. Is it possible that when a medical doctor says to you, "you have breast cancer. If you do not have surgery and start chemotherapy immediately, you will be dead in a year."

Is there any possibility that this could cause you to fear dying and trigger cancer in your lungs? And then you are diagnosed with metastatic lung cancer. Could this, therefore, be caused by the doctor's prognosis (outlook)?

Dr. Hamer believes that liver cancer is caused by what he called a 'starvation conflict'. One of the key functions of the liver is to develop digestive enzymes to digest food.

Is it possible that when you start taking chemotherapy and you vomit up everything you attempt to eat, your psyche concludes you are starving to death and increases the capacity of your liver to produce more digestive enzymes to try and stop you from starving to death? And then you are diagnosed with metastatic liver cancer. Could this be caused by the highly toxic chemotherapy making you vomit?

In the Germanic Healing Knowledge system, the lymphatic system is affected by a self-esteem conflict of an the inability to clean or remove an internal burden.

Is it possible that when you have a painful swelling on your breast, it would cause a self-esteem conflict of being unable to rid yourself of something unpleasant from your breast?

The lymphatic system closest to that organ is affected. Most commonly, it is the lymph nodes under the armpit next to the affected breast.

The lymph nodes reduce in size during the conflict, swell up, become painful, and are replenished during the second healing or repair phase.

You only become aware of the problem in the lymph glands once you have resolved the self-esteem conflict of having a painful swelling on your breast. This is typically either after the organ has healed or been removed via surgery.

It is at this point that medical doctors tell you the cancer has spread to your lymph nodes, a terrifying prognosis for any patient. Thrown into a panic that action must be taken immediately, rash medical decisions are too often made without question.

The swelling of the lymph gland next to the affected organ is merely a part of the healing process of the lymph gland. The lymph gland experiences ulceration, or tissue minus during the conflict of having a painful swelling on the organ.

Once the conflict has been resolved i.e. the pain in the organ has gone, the lymph glands start to heal. This involves pain and inflammation the same way the body heals when you cut your finger.

According to Dr. Hamer, it is biologically impossible for a mammary gland cell that has a biological program to create breast milk to swim through the bloodstream or lymphatic system and morph into a liver, lung, or lymphatic cell at the end of its swim.

If you put an apple seed in a pipe filled with human blood, what are the chances it will come out of the end of the pipe as an orange seed? Absurd, right? That is fundamentally what we are expected to believe with the metastasis hypothesis.

Treatment/Solution

Conventional Medicine

In CM, the treatment and solution is always a combination of surgery, chemotherapy, and radiation. The surgery will remove one breast. The chemotherapy will best case scenario make you infertile, and has a 98.5 percent likelihood of killing you.

According to a clinical oncology study carried out by oncologists in Australia in 2004, the five-year survival rate of patients who take chemotherapy for breast cancer have a 1.5% chance of surviving five years. Let that sink in.

The oncologists carrying out the study concluded:

"In an environment of scarce resources and cost-containment, there is a need for evidence-based assessment before any new or previously accepted treatment is accepted as standard practice.

To justify the continued funding and availability of drugs used in cytotoxic chemotherapy, a rigorous evaluation of the cost-effectiveness and impact on quality of life is urgently required."[2]

This clinical oncology study was subsequently buried.

Germanic Healing Knowledge

According to Dr. Hamer, the best way to solve a problem is a practical real-life resolution of the problem. With mammary gland cancer, this means you have to resolve the nest worry or care conflict that has triggered the biological program to start.

Once the biological program has achieved its biological purpose, it switches off naturally, it has achieved its biological purpose. The extra tissue or capacity is removed via natural fungi and tuberculosis bacteria in the body

If you have killed off your body's natural bacteria with heavy doses of antibiotics, the extra tissue can no longer be removed and will become an encapsulated cyst and remain.

With intraductal cancer, the most important first step is to identify the separation conflict that triggered the program that affected the milk ducts. Until you correctly identify the conflict that caused the problem to start, you cannot work out how to solve it. It is often very difficult to identify the cause of your problem on your own and you may want to consult a GHk consultant to help you with this process.

If you go to **https://danny-carroll.com/resources/** you will find references for GHk consultants to reach out to. It is critical to understand the exact cause of the problem, the moment in time when you experienced the separation conflict.

Working out your correct laterality, which way your brain is wired, is essential to make sure you have identified correctly whether it is your mother-child or partner breast that has been affected. Then you have to recall what was going on in your life when the problem started. The further back in time this happened, the more difficult it is to identify.

Once you work out what caused a problem to start, which is often the most difficult challenge, you can work out how to solve it. Solving the problem could come through a real-life resolution, or by changing the way you now view the problem.

Real-life resolutions are not always possible. For Dr. Hamer, it would have meant getting his wife pregnant. He suffered a testicular Teratoma when he was in his late 40s and had teenage children. His wife had passed her childbearing years. So a real-life practical resolution would have been very difficult for him, even if he had the knowledge at the time, which he didn't.

If your separation conflict was, for example, caused by a fight with a sibling because she took your favourite shoes without asking and destroyed them, after years of separation, it would be easy to look back on the fight and conclude that you have lost considerably more by not seeing your sibling for years than those shoes were ever worth.

Objectivity, forgiveness and understanding are very powerful tools to help resolve separation conflicts.

A general life tip. The amount of inflammation, pain and time any problem takes to heal is a multiplication of two factors. The length of time a conflict runs multiplied by how important the problem is to you determines what Dr. Hamer described as the "conflict mass."

The longer a problem runs, and the more important it is to you will determine how much fluid there is on the brain and organ, and the amount of time and pain you will have to go through for it to fully heal.

So two practical things you can do in life to make sure you never get seriously sick is whenever you have a problem, firstly, solve it as quickly as you can. Don't let problems drag on. And secondly, don't take life too seriously. The more important a problem is to you, the more intensely you experience the conflict, the greater the healing pain you will experience when you resolve the conflict, and the longer it will take to heal.

CHAPTER 6
HOW DO I SOLVE MY PROBLEM?

With the newly found knowledge you have acquired reading this digest, you now have a number of options of which path you want to follow to resolve your breast cancer issue.

From my experience, the most difficult challenge you currently face after reading this digest is getting your head around the idea that breast cancer is an integral part of nature's design and has a biological purpose or meaning.

We have been brainwashed all our lives to believe that cancer is a disease that spreads around your body and kills you from within. According to Dr. Hamer, that is utter rubbish.

Is there any possibility that our current medical system is a for-profit business that has weaponized nature by saying it is going wrong and you need to pay them hundreds of thousands of dollars to fix it, otherwise you will die, when nature is actually going right? Surely that cannot be the case. We all have to use our critical thinking skills and draw our own conclusions on this issue.

In the last report I read, the average cancer patient in the US is worth $1.5 million to the medical system. Money corrupts. And with that type of money to be made, it is a strong incentive to diagnose as many people as possible with cancer.

If you do a quick search online, you will find doctors who have been jailed for deliberately misdiagnosing patients with cancer. And it is just the tip of the iceberg.

The next challenge is to identify the conflict that caused breast cancer to start. In mammary gland cancer, this is relatively easy. The extra tissue (or tumor) will start growing as soon as you experience the nest worry or care conflict. In a short time after, you will be aware of it. In intraductal cancer, it can be more challenging as the separation conflict could have happened weeks, months or years before you become aware of it.

To make the challenge even more difficult, when we experience a traumatic event, our subconscious mind buries it. If we had every traumatic event we experienced in life in front of our conscious minds, we would be miserable. So the trauma that caused the problem may not be immediately accessible to your conscious mind.

To solve this problem, you may need to consult family members and close friends to piece together what happened to get the memory of the experience to surface in your conscious mind.

Mammary Gland Cancer

With mammary gland cancer, the most important thing to focus on is to resolve the nest worry or care conflict that triggered the biological program to start. The mammary glands will continue to produce milk and be diagnosed as lobular cancer whilst the nest worry or care conflict continues.

Once the conflict has been resolved, the biological program will switch off and the extra tissue added during the conflict will be naturally removed by fungi and tuberculosis mycobacteria, if you still have them. If you do not, the lump will be encapsulated and stay in the breast.

Throughout the conflict, it is advisable to either get a partner to suckle the milk from the breast, or get a breast pump and evacuate it. This will help to remove the inflammation and pressure inside the breast, and of course, this is nature's design.

If you do not do this, the breast will become small and hard at the end of the healing process. This is not a health risk, but is not aesthetically pleasing.

You will feel exhausted and have zero energy during the healing process. Expect this and do not fight it. If your body needs rest, it is advisable to listen to it. If you fight it, you will just extend the length of the healing process.

You will also wake up in the night in puddles of sweat. This is called night sweats and happens when tuberculosis mycobacteria is removing the extra tissue added to your mammary glands. Keep plenty of water at your bedside. You will wake up in the night incredibly thirsty.

If the breast does break open, you will have to learn to live with the putrid smell of flesh rotting until it heals. This is very unpleasant. I had cancer in my jaw in 2019 and had both the taste and smell of rotting flesh in my mouth for four months. So I have personal experience of this. That too in my mouth and sinuses. Most important is to have a high protein diet to replace the protein-rich fluids that will leak from the open wound.

Intraductal Breast Cancer

With intraductal breast cancer, if the breast is swollen and painful, it means you have resolved the separation conflict that caused the problem. The swelling and inflammation in ductal cancer only start after you have resolved the separation conflict.

If you consciously connect the original separation conflict trauma, and the intraductal cancer symptoms, it will trigger a cathartic healing process. This is almost impossible to both explain and understand until you have experienced it. Just say to yourself, 'I know the milk ducts in my breast are swollen because I resolved the separation conflict with (fill in the blanks), it will accelerate the healing process. You have nothing to lose by trying it.

It is recommended that you evacuate any fluid build-up in the breast by either getting a partner to suckle the breast or by using a breast pump. Evacuating the fluid will help to reduce the inflammation and take some of the pressure out of the swollen breast. It will also prevent the breast from becoming small and hard at the end of the healing process.

Evacuating the fluid from the breast will be painful at the beginning due to the blockage in the milk ducts. It is easier to moderate this pain by getting someone to suckle the breast than using a breast pump.

Try putting a savoy cabbage leaf on the breast under your bra. This will help to soften the breast and reduce inflammation. You can also try using "milking grease" on the breast to help keep it soft.

When the itching starts you can use a cream with a local anaesthetic on the outside of the breast to reduce the itching. There is nothing you can do about the itching inside the milk ducts. Similar to when you cut your finger, this itching is a necessary evil and something you will have to push on through. If you scratch the breast to relieve the itching, it will just make it worse.

If the nipple is inverted and either the breast is numb, or the skin has started flaking on the breast, it means that you have an unresolved separation conflict still running. You have two choices. You can either not resolve the conflict and live with the status quo. Or you can work on resolving the conflict with the understanding that when you resolve it, the breast will become swollen and painful for some time.

If you decide to resolve the conflict, the guidance above on milking the breast and applying a savoy cabbage leaf under your bra and milking grease would apply.

Be prepared to either suffer from short-term memory loss, or even faint and pass out. This is part of the healing crisis and the way nature removes fluid from your organ and brain. If you expect this to happen, it does not cause any fear when it happens.

It is best to advise those closest to you that this is could happen and advise them not to disturb you or attempt to wake you up. If you disturb the process, it will keep repeating until the fluid is removed.

This may also happen without you being aware of it. Most often it will happen at 4 am whilst you are sleeping, but it can also happen during the daytime so it is best to be prepared in case it does happen during waking hours.

I will finish this digest with a case study of ductal carcinoma experience provided by a student of Germanic Healing Knowledge. It gives a practical demonstration of how you can go through the process of healing the breast from a separation conflict without fear and how the process can be managed peacefully.

I have been studying German New Medicine for a few years. It is wonderful to see again and again how exactly it functions, in my own case, my family, for my friends or acquaintances.

My children, who grew up with this awareness, know quite well how to deal with health challenges. When they experience a conflict, it is normally resolved quickly. They come to me and say: "Mama, I know exactly why I had the cough or the cold" or "why my knee hurts"...

And when at times a conflict cannot be resolved immediately, then they come meekly: "Mama, can I talk to you later?" It is pleasing to see how the children are growing up with a different understanding of "illness". That are anyway mostly healing phases.

I cannot protect myself or my children against conflicts. We are all responsible for how we deal with conflicts. However, we have learned to deal with conflicts differently.

We all have baggage and carry around unresolved conflicts. I was lugging around such a conflict for ten years, without actually being aware of it.

I have been happily married for 13 years and have two daughters. It was always my most ardent wish to have one more child, a son. My husband, the sole earner, did not agree with having a third child. I always quietly believed that if I got pregnant and we had a third child, he would have been very happy. So I hung on to the desire.

I did not believe in taking the contraceptive pill or using protection during intercourse so there was always a chance I would get pregnant. Each time I thought I could be pregnant, I took a pregnancy test. Each time, I was disappointed when the test was negative. I was preoccupied with it for a couple of days, and then I forgot about it. I never said a word about this to my husband.

Recently there was such a situation once again. As usual, I took a test, however this time I was not at all surprised by the result - quite the contrary. I thought to myself: "You are now 37 years old and practically too old to have another child. The children are growing up and now to begin all over again - no, you really do not want that anymore!"

A few days later, I felt that my left breast (I am right-handed) hurt a lot, it was extremely sensitive. The next day, I noticed that a red mark had formed. The breast was hot, cancer red, severely swollen, and felt hard. Even the mammilla had pulled inward (retracted). I did not panic, for I really knew, that this could "only" be the healing phase of a separation conflict and a so-called mammary ductal "carcinoma".

But I was worried that I was not clear about the conflict that caused it. It could only be a separation conflict from my mother or my child. But there was no such conflict in sight. It is extremely important for me to find out what the conflict was, and how long it lasted so that I could understand the intensity and duration of the conflict, so I knew what to expect in the healing phase.

I tried quark compresses that have a cooling effect, to counteract the swelling, and also placed ice packs on the relevant spot on the breast. But the next morning the redness and even the swelling had increased. The redness had now spread around the breast eight to nine centimeters, however, the pain was bearable. Now and then I felt severe twitches, which were very uncomfortable. I also had the impression that the breast had become externally deformed and rubbery.

I subsequently rubbed in milking grease and massaged gently up to the mammilla.

And I noticed something else: my short-term memory was affected. The quark compresses I used for a total of five days, however only at night, and during the day I stuck ice packs or cold sheets in a larger bra. After six days, the redness had reduced a bit, though the breast was still thick, hard, and heavy, and the mammilla remained retracted.

In all my deliberations, I asked myself: What is the mother-child separation conflict I have resolved? In the process, I thought about the situation regarding the pregnancy test, but that seemed to be too abstract to me, too far-fetched. I was not sure.

Finally, I confided in an acquaintance, who is also well informed about German New Medicine. However, she was of the opinion that it could only be this problem. After consultation with "headquarters", she also confirmed this opinion. And it was actually not as abstract as it initially seemed. For I had, even if just mentally, finally separated from my "son". It is difficult for most to imagine that a problem like this could be triggered as a result.

So how did it go from then on? The acquaintance suggested that I replace the quark compresses with compresses of cabbage leaves. I remembered that my father had earlier used them quite often for some aches and pains and had also been successful. And so the suggestion was not really odd for me, as it may sound to some.

Anyhow, the cabbage always had great standing in ancient times and was nearly a universal remedy. It is said that the Romans did not know any other "remedy" for six centuries. They used it as an internal and external cleaning agent, for compresses, and for treatment of wounds of their legionaries.

I procured a very fresh, green, juicy savoy cabbage. In the evening, I broke off a few leaves, washed them thoroughly, cut the thick ribs out and rolled them out flat with a rolling pin.

Then I distributed them on my breast and to retain the moisture, I placed another film on them. The next morning the surface of the breast initially looked quite wizened. However, after a while, it looked smoother again. The redness had disappeared, the tenseness had somewhat reduced, and I even believed - or imagined - the breast had become a bit smaller. I continued with these compresses and left the cabbage leaves for up to twelve hours or more to take effect.

After a few days, I was happy to see that the breast had actually become smaller and even softer. I was quite happy when I saw that even the mammilla gradually curved outwards again. Likewise, the stings in the breast were reduced. But for that, now there was a terrible itch.

In any case, I continued the procedure for a while and rubbed milking grease into the breast regularly, and of course, continued to cool. In the meantime, everything regressed again.

The whole process lasted a total of three weeks.

It is impossible to imagine what would have happened to me if I had not already known about German New Medicine. Probably I would have been operated on by now, the breast perhaps amputated and totally mutilated.

When you learn that breast cancer is not a disease, and cancer does not spread around your body like some foreign invading army, it changes your outlook on the problem.

The understanding that breast cancer is a part of nature's design to help you to nurture a sick loved one, or evacuate the milk from the breast when you are separated from a loved one, changes your outlook on the problem and how you approach solving it.

Given the alternative is going to a medical doctor, having your breast removed by surgery, which anyway does not solve the problem as the breast cancer biological program runs in the brain and not the organ, and taking chemotherapy that you have a 1.5% of surviving, if you follow nature's design, you have a far better chance of achieving a positive outcome, in my experience.

We are all responsible for our health, or lack thereof. I take decisions on the path I think is best to fully recover my health when I face health challenges. And I do quite often.

Learning Germanic Healing Knowledge does not stop you from getting into conflicts in life, but it helps tremendously to work out how best to resolve the conflicts and manage the symptoms of the process.

But there is not one path to follow, everybody's paths are different. You have to take decisions based on what you think is best for you.

Best of luck on your healing journey.

CHAPTER 7
THE MONTHLY DIGEST

Every month, I will explore one disease and compare its cause(s) and proposed solutions from a Conventional Medicine and a Germanic New Medicine/ Germanische Heilkunde perspective. You can sign up for this at my website **https://danny-carrol l.com.**

When you sign up, you will receive a **free 400+ page GNM lexicon** that lists the 'causes' of almost every known disease, and includes over 500 case examples. Plus, a **FREE One-Year Course** of 6–7-minute MP3 daily classes to start learning Germanic Healing Knowledge.

If there is a specific health challenge you are facing and would like me to cover it, please email me with a short description of your situation. I will prioritize the health issues I write about based on the greatest need.

Finally, if you found value in this short book, I would greatly appreciate it if you could leave a review. As an independent author and publisher, book reviews help tremendously, even just one or two lines.

Most importantly, share your stories about resolving your breast cancer. These testimonials are always a great encouragement to others who are only a few steps behind you on the path to taking charge of their own health. Also, I love the goose-bumps I get when I read them.

Link for leaving a review (tht.fyi/bc)

Best of luck on your healing journey.

ABOUT THE AUTHOR

Danny spent the first half of his life living in London, UK, and completed his education with a master's degree from the London School of Economics. He moved to live and work in India in the mid-1990s.

Danny has spent the last 20 years studying alternative healing therapies in search of the Holy Grail of health and wellness. Following a cathartic healing experience in 2012, he has focused on mind-body healing protocols for the last 10 years.

Danny is not a doctor, but he has been blessed with a curious, questioning mind, and an abundance of critical thinking skills. He has a very pragmatic approach to life and his philosophy is, "If it works, use it." He is very comfortable exploring new ideas and healing protocols that most, for some reason, are unwilling to explore... until they have no other alternative.

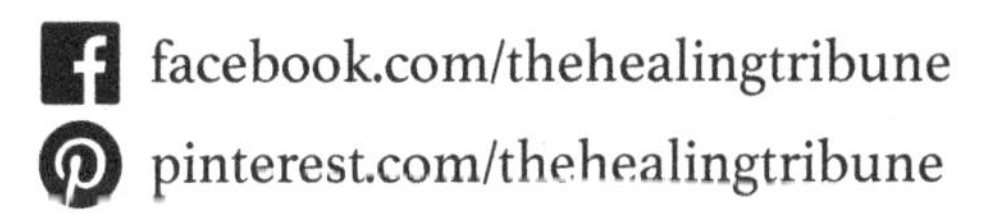

ENDNOTES

5. Danny's Comments and Observations

1. https://www.ncbi.nlm.nih.gov/pmc/articles/PMC5385482/
2. https://danny-carroll.com/content/docs/Clinical-Oncology-Study.pdf

L - #0218 - 071123 - C0 - 216/140/6 - PB - DID3756546